THE ULTIMATE REVOLUTIONARY OF THE CANCER CODE:

Tips on surviving a cancer adventure

Bobbie W. Lewis

Table of content

AF416498

Understanding Cancer Risk

 Risk is the chance that an event will be. When talking about cancer, the threat is most frequently used to describe the chance that a person will get cancer. It's also used to describe the chance that cancer will come back or reoccur.
Experimenters and croakers use cancer threats to ameliorate the health of numerous people. One illustration of this is understanding the pitfalls of smoking. Scientists discovered that smoking increases the threat of lung cancer. They used this knowledge to launch a global anti-smoking crusade to help save lives.

Understanding threat factors

A cancer threat factor is anything that increases a person's chance of getting cancer. Yet most threat factors don't directly cause cancer. Some people with several threat factors norway develop cancer. And others with no known threat factors do.

It's important to know your threat factors and talk about them with your health care platoon. It'll help you make better life choices to ameliorate your health. This information could also help your croaker decide if you need inheritable testing and comforting(see below).

General threat factors for cancer include
Aged age
A particular or family history of cancer
Using tobacco
rotundity
Alcohol
Some types of viral infections, similar as mortal papillomavirus(HPV)
Specific chemicals
Exposure to radiation, including ultraviolet radiation from the sun

You can avoid some threat factors by stopping parlous actions. These include using tobacco and alcohol, being fat, and getting multiple sunburns. Other threat factors can not be avoided, similar to getting aged. These factors will be explained more in the coming chapter.

Threat factors and cancer webbing
Understanding your threat for cancer can help your croaker decide whether you could profit from; A cancer webbing test, similar to a mammogram or colonoscopy. A webbing test at an earlier age and more frequently than routine webbing. Surgery or drug to lower your cancer threat
For illustration, a woman whose mama had bone cancer is at least doubly as likely to have bone cancer than a woman who doesn't have the same family history. Some women have strong family histories or inheritable mutations linked to bone cancer. Since they're at a veritably high threat of bone cancer, they may choose to remove

their guts to help cancer. This surgery appears to lower the threat of getting bone cancer by at least 95. Also, these women may choose to take a drug to lower the threat of bone cancer.

People with a strong family history of cancer may consider inheritable testing. Your croaker or inheritable counselor can talk with you about getting certain inheritable tests. They can tell you your threat of getting cancer grounded on your family history and other threat factors.

Understanding the difference between an absolute and relative threat

Croakers use absolute threat and relative threat to assess if a person's threat is advanced or lower than that of either the general population or a certain group of people.

The absolute threat is the chance that a person will develop a complaint during a given time. This identifies how numerous people are at threat of a complaint in the general population.

For a case, consider the statement " 1 out of 8 women(12.5) will get bone cancer in her continuance. " This describes the absolute threat to the general population of women. It can not identify the threat to a certain person or group of people. For illustration, an absolute threat can not show if a group of aged women has an advanced threat of bone cancer than a group of young women.

Relative threat compares the threat of complaint between two groups of people. It compares one group with a certain threat factor for a complaint to another group's threat.

For a case, imagine you're comparing the threat of bone cancer among 2 groups of 100 women. But only the women in 1 group have a certain threat factor for bone cancer. The other group of women doesn't have this threat factor. Experimenters keep track of how numerous people from each group develop cancer over a certain time.

Let's say they find that 2 women who have the same threat factor get cancer. But only 1 woman without this threat factor gets cancer. Also, those in the first group have 2 times the threat of the alternate group. This is a 100% increase in relative threat. The absolute threat, still, would be 2 or 2 out of 100 people.

Cases can use threat measures to make better choices about life changes or cancer webbing. It's also important to know the difference between absolute and relative threats. For example, the relative threat in the last illustration might sound high. It linked a person's relative threat of developing cancer by 100.

But look at the absolute threat to get a more complete picture. That is, 1 person in 100 compared to 2 people in 100. Still, make sure you find the absolute threat If you want to compare the exploration you hear about in the news to your situation. utmost exploration studies report relative pitfalls. This can make the threat sound more advanced than it actually is. This will be explained plainly in the coming sub-content; general order of threat.

Questions to ask your health care platoon

Statistical language can be hard to understand. So ask your health care platoon to explain what this information means in your situation. Consider bringing up these questions about the cancer threat

What threat factors do I have? How do they affect my threat of cancer?

What's my chance of developing cancer in the coming 5 times? In my continuance?

What can I do to lower my threat of cancer?

What if I change my geste to exclude a threat factor(for illustration, quit smoking or lose weight)? Also, what are my chances of getting cancer in the coming 5 times? In my continuance?

What if I find out about a new threat factor, similar to a relative developing cancer? Also, how important does the threat increase?

What cancer webbing tests do you recommend? How frequently should I've them?

Cancer threat What the figures mean

Take the time to understand what cancer threat is and how it's measured. This can help you put your own cancer threat into perspective.

You might wonder about your chances of developing cancer. News reports can make it sound as if the everyday commodity is set up to dramatically raise your threat. Sorting through all the information and figuring out what is valid can be tricky.

When scientists talk about threat, they are pertaining to a probability — the chance that a commodity may do, but not a guarantee that it will. For illustration, if you flip a coin, there's one chance in two, or a 50 percent chance, that the coin will land heads up.
Threat estimates for cancer and other conditions are determined by studying large groups of people. Experimenters concentrate on the probability that any person or order of people will develop the complaint over a certain period of time. They also look to see what characteristics or actions are associated with the increased or dropped threat.

The general order of threat
The threat is generally divided into two orders: absolute threat and relative threat.

Absolute threat
Absolute threat refers to the factual numeric chance or probability of developing cancer during a specified time period — for illustration, within the time, within the coming five times, by age 50, by age 70, or during the course of a continuance.

One type of absolute threat is continuance threat, which is the probability that an existent will develop cancer during the course of a continuance. For case, an American man's absolute threat of developing prostate cancer in his continuance is about 12 percent. Put another way, about 12 out of every 100 men will develop prostate cancer at some time in their lives. This also means that 88 out of every 100 men will not develop prostate cancer.

Continuance threat is not the threat that a person will develop cancer in the coming time or the coming five times. An existent's cancer threat has a lot to do with other factors, similar to age. For case, an American woman's continuance threat of developing colon and rectal cancer is about 4 percent, or about 40 out of every,000 women. But her threat of developing colon and rectal cancer before the age of 50 is 0.4 percent, or about 4 out of every,000 women.

Relative threat
Relative threat gives you a comparison or rate rather than an absolute value. It shows the strength of the relationship between a threat factor and a particular type of cancer by comparing the number of cancers in a group of people who have a particular particularity with the number of cancers in a group of people who do not have that particularity.

For a case, compare the relative lung cancer threat for people who bomb with the relative lung cancer threat in an analogous group of people who do not bomb. You might hear relative threats being expressed like this The threat of lung cancer for smokers is 25 times more advanced than the threat for people who do not bomb. So the relative threat of lung cancer for smokers is 25.

A relative threat is also given a chance. For illustration, the threat of lung cancer for smokers is,500 percent more advanced than it's for people who do not bomb.
When you hear about a relative threat, there is no upper limit to the chance of an increase in threat. The utmost people suppose 100 percent is the loftiest possible threat, but that is not true in this case.

A relative threat of 100 percent means your threat is doubly as high as that of someone without that threat factor. A 200 percent relative threat means that you're three times as likely to develop that condition.

The threat seems lesser when put in these terms. A 100 percent increase in threat may feel enormous, but if the threat began as 1 in 100 people, a 100 percent increase in threat means that 2 out of 100 will be affected.

Where do cancer threat statistics come from?
utmost information about cancer threat and threat factors comes from studies that concentrate on large, well-defined groups of people. Cancer experimenters have linked numerous of the major environmental factors that contribute to cancer, including smoking for lung cancer and sun for skin cancer. Uncovering more subtle cancer pitfalls has proved more delicate.

numerous studies of cancer threat factors calculate on experimental approaches. In these studies, experimenters keep track of a group of people several times without trying to change their lives or give them special treatment. This can help scientists find out who develops a complaint, what those people have in common, and how they differ from those who did not get sick.
How do cancer threat statistics relate to me?
Threat statistics can be frustrating because they can not tell you your threat of cancer. Studies may have set up that American men have about a 40 percent chance of developing cancer in their continuances, but that does not mean your threat is 40 percent if you are a man. Your individual threat is grounded on numerous different factors, such as age and habits(including eating habits), family history of cancer, and the terrain in which you live.

Indeed also, the combination of threat factors might not apply to you. Cancer is individualistic. You can have two people with the same age, coitus, race, socio- profitable status, and relative cultures and still have different guests. threat statistics are helpful in general statements similar as" exercising regularly coincides with a reduced threat of habitual conditions, similar to cancer." But exercising regularly will not guarantee that you will not get cancer.

Talk with your croaker
about your threat of cancer. He or she can review what rudiments in your life may increase your threat. You can also bandy about what to do to help lower this threat.

Keep cancer threat statistics in perspective

You might hear a news report about a study that seems to indicate you may be at increased threat of a particular type of cancer. Do not jump to conclusions grounded on this one report. Take a step back and suppose about what the threat really means.

experimental studies are not reliable. Experimenters agree that one study by itself is not authoritative. This is why you occasionally see studies with putatively antithetical results.

Scientists weigh the substantiation of numerous exploration studies over time to determine whether a finding is true. News reports, however, concentrate on each new study in insulation, rather than as a part of an evolving picture. This can occasionally beget gratuitous alarm or confusion.

When you read or see a report about cancer threat statistics, pay attention to these details

Who is being observed? A news report may say a certain exertion increases the threat of cancer for a group of people. But who was being observed in the study? Pay attention to the periods of the people and their characteristics. For example, some people are genetically fitted for certain types of cancer.

How many people were studying? In general, studies involving thousands of people are more accurate than those that examine a small group of people.

Have analogous studies been done? The findings of one study are more dependable if they are analogous to the findings of other studies. occasionally, the study was not carried out enough times to make it statistically significant.

News reports that focus on intimidating statistics, similar to a 300 percent increase in threat, but do not give you an environment are not helpful. However, gather further information and talk to your croaker, if you are concerned about the threat.

Chapter 2: Causes of Cancer

Cancer is a condition developed in the mortal body in which some cells grow out of control and spread to other corridors of the body. Cancer can begin in any of the billions of cells that make up one Homo sapiens. mortal cells typically divide and multiply to induce new cells as demanded by the body. When cells come too old or damaged to serve, they die and are replaced by new bones.
This ordered process occasionally can break down, performing in abnormal or damaged cells growing and multiplying when they should not. These cells can grow into excrescences, which are towel lumps. Excrescences can be benign or cancerous(benign).
Cancerous excrescences can attack hard healthy napkins and spread to other corridors of the body, performing in the conformation of new excrescences(a process called metastasis). nasty excrescences are another name for cancerous excrescences. numerous cancers form solid excrescences, but leukemia similar to cancers of the blood generally does not.
Benign excrescences don't access or spread into girding napkins. Benign excrescences infrequently reappear after being removed, although nasty excrescences do every so frequently. Still, benign excrescences can grow to be extremely enormous. Some, similar to benign brain excrescences, can produce serious symptoms or indeed be murderous.

Threat Factors For Cancer

It's delicate to identify why one existent develops cancer while another does not. Certain threat factors, still, have been demonstrated to raise a person's chances of growing cancer in exploration studies. There are other factors associated with reduced cancer threat.

occasionally these are pertained to as defensive threat factors or simply defensive factors.

 Chemical or other substance exposure, as well as certain actions, are all cancer threat factors. They also include factors that people have no control over, similar to age and family history. A family history of some malice may indicate the presence of an inherited cancer pattern.
The maturity of cancer threat factors is first discovered in epidemiological studies. Scientists examine wide groups of people in these examinations and compare those who acquire cancer to those who do not. These studies may reveal that persons who acquire cancer are more or less likely than those who don't develop cancer to bear in specific ways or be exposed to certain substances.

 Causes of Cancer
 The following is a list of the most well-studied known or suspected cancer threat factors. While some of these threat factors, similar to getting aged, perhaps can be avoided, others can not. Limiting your exposure to preventable threat factors may help you avoid some excrescences.
Rotundity fat people are more likely to develop cancers of the bone(in women who have gone through menopause), colon, rectum, endometrium(uterine filling), esophagus, order, pancreas, and gallbladder. Consuming a good diet, being physically active, and maintaining a healthy weight, on the other hand, may help minimize the threat of certain cancers. Other diseases, such as heart complaints, type II diabetes, and high blood pressure, can be reduced by espousing these good habits.

 Any cancer treatment can be employed as the first line of defense, still, surgery is the most common original cancer treatment for the most current cancers.

Tobacco The operation of tobacco is a major cause of cancer and cancer-related mortality. Because tobacco products and unresistant smoking include numerous chemicals that disrupt DNA, those who use tobacco products or are regularly exposed to ambient tobacco banks(also known as a secondary bank) have an advanced threat of cancer.

Tobacco use causes lung cancer, tracheal cancer, mouth cancer, esophageal cancer, throat cancer, bladder cancer, order cancer, liver cancer, stomach cancer, pancreas cancer, colon and rectum cancer, and cervical cancer, as well as acute myeloid leukemia. Smokeless tobacco druggies(snuff or biting tobacco) had an advanced threat of mouth, esophageal, and pancreatic cancers.

There can be no similar claim as a " safe cigarette consumption position ". People who use tobacco products of any kind are laboriously encouraged to quit. People who quit smoking, anyhow of age, have a much longer life expectancy than those who continue to bomb. The smoking conclusion at the time of a cancer opinion also lowers the threat of mortality.

Consuming redundant alcohol increases your chances of developing cancers of the mouth, throat, esophagus, larynx(voice box), liver, and bone cancer. The more you drink, the more advanced your threat. Those who drink alcohol and bank tobacco have a mainly increased threat of cancer.

According to croakers, people who drink should do it in temperance. According to the civil government's Dietary Guidelines for Americans, moderate alcohol consumption is defined as one drink per day for women and two drinks per day for men.

Certain factors of red wine, similar to resveratrol, have been claimed to have anti-cancer characteristics. There's no substantiation, still, that consuming red wine lowers the threat of cancer.

Habitual Inflammation Inflammation is a normal physiological response that assists in the mending of a wounded towel. When a damaged towel releases chemicals, the seditious process begins. White blood cells respond by producing chemicals that beget cells to divide and increase in order to help repair the detriment. The seditious process will be over once the crack is healed.

The seditious process in habitual inflammation can start indeed if there's no injury, and it doesn't terminate when it should. It isn't always clear why the inflammation persists. Infections that don't go down, adverse vulnerable responses to normal napkins, and factors like rotundity can all induce habitual inflammation. The seditious response can damage the DNA and can ultimately lead to cancer. People with habitual seditious intestinal diseases like ulcerative colitis and Crohn's complaint are more likely to develop colon cancer.

 Age Factor The major threat factor for cancer in general, as well as for numerous specific cancer types, is growing age. Overall, cancer prevalence rates rise constantly with age, from smaller than 25 cases per,000 people in age groups under 20 to around 350 cases per,000 people in age groups 45 – 49, and further than,000 cases per,000 people in age groups 60 and aged.

According to utmost recent statistical exploration data, the typical age of a cancer opinion is 66 times. This means that half of the cancer cases are in those under the age of 50 times, and the other half in people over 50 times. numerous common cancer types borrow an analogous pattern. Bone cancer, for illustration, has a median age of 62 times, while colorectal cancer has a median age of 67 times, lung cancer has a median age of 71 times, and prostate cancer has a typical age of 66 times.

 Radiation Ionizing radiation is a type of radiation that has enough energy to damage DNA and cause cancer. Radon,x-rays, gamma shafts, and other high-energy radiation are exemplifications of ionizing radiation. People haven't been set up to get cancer from lower-energy,non-ionizing kinds of radiation, similar to visible light and the energy from cell phones.

X-rays, gamma shafts, nascence patches, beta patches, and neutrons are exemplifications of high-energy radiation that can damage DNA and cause cancer. These types of radiation can be emitted in nuclear power factory accidents as well as during the development, testing, and use of infinitesimal munitions.

Casket-rays, reckoned tomography(CT) reviews, positron emigration tomography(PET) reviews, and radiation remedies are all examples of medical procedures that might damage cells and lead to cancer.

Still, the chances of developing cancer as a result of these medical treatments are extremely low. Whereas the benefits always exceed the hazards, colorful ionizing radiations similar to nascence, beta, and gamma shafts are performed to treat colorful types of excrescences in optimal conditions.

Contagious Agents Contagions, bacteria, and spongers, among other contagious agents, can beget cancer or raise the threat of cancer development. Some contagions can intrude with the signaling that regulates cell growth and proliferation. Likewise, some infections compromise the vulnerable system, leaving the system susceptible to other cancer-causing conditions. habitual inflammation, which can lead to cancer, is also caused by some contagions, bacteria, and spongers.
 The maturity of contagions associated with an elevated threat of cancer can be transmitted from one person to another via blood and/ or other fleshly fluids. By getting vaccinated, not having sexual intercourse, and not participating in needles, you can reduce your threat of infection.

 HIV(Human Immunodeficiency Syndrome)- The contagion that causes an acquired immunodeficiency pattern(AIDS) is HIV- AIDS. HIV infection doesn't beget cancer, but it weakens the vulnerable system and makes the body less suitable to fight off other cancer-causing ails. HIV infection increases the threat of several cancers, including Kaposi sarcoma, tubercles(including non-Hodgkin carcinoma and Hodgkin complaint), and cancers of the cervix, anus, lung, liver, and throat.

Immunosuppression numerous people who have gone through organ transplants are given medicines to suppress their vulnerable systems so that the organ won't be rejected by the body. These " immunosuppressive " specifics weaken the vulnerable system's capability to descry and destroy cancer cells as well as repel cancer-causing infections. HIV infection affects the vulnerable system and increases the chance of developing certain malice.
 Transplant donors have an elevated threat of a variety of malice, according to exploration. contagious pathogens can beget some of these excrescences, but not all of them. Non-Hodgkin carcinoma(NHL) and malice of the lung, order, and liver are the four most common cancers among transplant cases, and they occur more constantly in these people than in the overall population. NHL is caused by the Epstein- Barr contagion(EBV), whereas liver cancer is caused by habitual hepatitis B(HBV) and hepatitis C(HCV)

contagion infection. Cancers of the lungs and feathers aren't known to be linked to infection.

Gene Mutations The finding of particular types of genes that play a part in cancer has been a huge step forward in cancer exploration. Over 90 excrescences are set up to contain some form of inheritable mutation. Some of these changes are heritable, while others are arbitrary, indicating they are spontaneous or as a result of exposure to the terrain(generally over numerous times).

Types of Cancer Genes
The following are three primary types of genes that can affect cell development and are altered(shifted) in specific types of cancers

Tumor Suppressor Genes These genes can descry indecorous cell development and reduplication, similar to cancer cells, and can stop them from reproducing until the insufficiency is repaired.
Oncogenes The healthy growth of cells is regulated by these genes.
Mismatch- Repair Genes When DNA is replicated to produce a new cell, these genes help decry crimes. These genes repair the mismatch and amend the error if the DNA doesn't " match " precisely.

Cancer-Causing Substances Changes in specific genes fully change the way our cells medium, which causes cancer. When DNA is replicated throughout the cell division process, some of these inheritable variations are natural. Others, still, are caused by DNA damage caused by environmental factors. Substances, similar to those set up in cigarette banks, or radiation, similar to UV shafts from the sun, are exemplifications of these types of exposures.

Some cancer-causing exposures, similar to cigarette banks and the sun's shafts, can be avoided. Other poisons, on the other hand, are more delicate to avoid, particularly if they're present in the air we breathe, the water we drink, the food we consume, or the accouterments we use in our jobs.
Scientists are looking at whether types of exposures may beget or contribute to cancer growth. People may be suitable to avoid dangerous exposures if they understand what they will be and where they can be set up.

Aflatoxins, Arsenic, Beryllium, liquid Silica, Formaldehyde, Nickel- composites, Thorium, and Wood Dust are the most likely carcinogens to affect mortal health.

numerous cancers, according to utmost experts, can be averted or the chance of getting excrescences can be significantly dropped. Some of the ways are straightforward, while others are more extreme, depending on one's perspective. The simplest strategy for precluding cancer is to avoid its implicit causes.

Parting(or better yet, norway starting) smoking is at the top of utmost croakers' and experimenters ' dockets. numerous chemicals and venoms, as well as extreme sun(by reducing exposure or using sunscreen), are good strategies to avoid cancer.

Some malice can be avoided by avoiding contact with certain contagions and other infections. People who work in close proximity to cancer-causing agents(druggists, X-ray technicians, ionizing radiation experimenters, asbestos workers) should take all necessary safety precautions.

Chapter 3: Fatigue and Weakness

What's Fatigue or Weakness?
Fatigue and weakness are frequently used to describe the same thing. But they actually are different.

Weakness
Weakness is when strength is dropped and redundant trouble is demanded to move a certain part of the body or the entire body. Weakness is due to loss of muscle strength. Weakness can be a big part of why cancer cases feel fatigued.

Fatigue
Fatigue is an extreme feeling of frazzle or lack of energy, frequently described as being exhausted. Fatigue is a commodity that lasts

indeed when a person seems to be getting enough sleep. It can have numerous causes, including working too much, having disturbed sleep, stress and solicitude, not having enough physical exertion, and going through an illness and its treatment.

The fatigue that frequently comes with cancer is called cancer-related fatigue. It's veritably common. Between 80 and 100 people with cancer report having fatigue. The fatigue felt by people with cancer is different from the fatigue of diurnal life and different from the tired feeling people might flashback having before they had cancer.

People with cancer might describe it as feeling veritably weak, lackadaisical, drained, or " washed out " that may drop for a while but also comes back. Some may feel too tired to eat, walk to the restroom, or indeed use the television remote. It can be hard to suppose or move. Rest might help for a short time but doesn't make it go down, and just a little exertion can be exhausting. For some people with cancer, this kind of fatigue causes further torture than pain, nausea, puking, or depression.

What causes fatigue and weakness?
In people with cancer, weakness might be caused by having and recovering from surgery, low blood counts or low electrolyte(blood chemistry) situations, infection, or changes in hormone situations.

Still, the causes of cancer-related fatigue are frequently harder to determine because there are frequently numerous factors involved. It might be from cancer itself and/ or a side effect of the cancer treatment. How cancer and treatment might beget fatigue isn't well understood, but some possible reasons are

Cancer and cancer treatment can change normal protein and hormone situations that are linked to seditious processes which can beget or worsen fatigue.
Treatments kill normal cells and cancer cells, which leads to a figure-up of cell waste. Your body uses redundant energy to clean up and repair damaged towels.

Cancer forms poisonous substances in the body that change the way normal cells work.

Besides direct goods of cancer and its treatment, people with cancer frequently also witness other effects that can add together to increase fatigue. These are effects like surgery, stress and solicitude, changes in exertion position, and changes in blood counts, electrolytes, and hormone situations.

Fatigue that's due to cancer and its treatment can last for weeks, months, or times. It frequently continues after treatment ends.

For people who have surgery for cancer with no other treatment, fatigue frequently decreases or goes down over time as they recover from surgery.

For people getting chemotherapy, targeted remedy, or immunotherapy in cycles, fatigue frequently gets worse at first and may get better until the coming treatment, when the pattern starts again.

For those getting radiation remedies, fatigue generally gets worse as the treatment goes on and frequently lessens within many months after treatment is complete.

Fatigue can differ from one day to the coming in how bad it's and how important it bothers you

Be inviting and make it hard for you to feel well

Make it hard for you to be with your musketeers and family

Make it hard for you to do effects you typically do, including going to work

Make it harder for you to follow your cancer treatment plan.

What to look for

You feel tired and it doesn't get better with rest or sleep, it keeps coming back, or it becomes severe.

You're more tired than usual during or after exertion.

You're feeling tired and it's not related to exertion.

You're too tired to do the effects you typically do.

Your arms and legs feel heavy and hard to move.
You have no energy.
You feel veritably weak.
You spend further time in bed and/ or sleep further. Or, you may have trouble sleeping.
You stay in bed for more than 24 hours.
You come confused or can't concentrate or concentrate on your studies.
Your frazzle disrupts your work, social life, or daily routine.
It may be hard for you to talk about it, but tell your cancer care platoon about your fatigue. Tell them how it's affecting your life. Someone in your platoon should be suitable to help you if they know you're having this problem. Managing fatigue is part of good cancer care. Work with your cancer care platoon to find and treat the causes of your fatigue.

Chapter4: Prevention is the cure

Cancer forestallment 7 tips to reduce your threat
Concerned about cancer forestallment? Take charge by making changes similar to eating a healthy diet and getting regular wireworks.
You've presumably heard clashing reports about cancer forestallment. occasionally specific cancer- forestallment tips recommended in one study are advised against in another.
Frequently, what is known about cancer forestallment is still evolving. Still, it's well-accepted that your chances of developing cancer are affected by the life choices you make.
So if you are interested in precluding cancer, take comfort in the fact that simple life changes can make a difference. Consider these cancer- forestallment tips.

1. Do not use tobacco
Using any type of tobacco puts you on a collision course with cancer. Smoking has been linked to colorful types of cancer — including cancer of the lung, mouth, throat, larynx, pancreas,

bladder, cervix, and order. Biting tobacco has been linked to cancer of the oral depression and pancreas. Indeed if you do not use tobacco, exposure to the secondary banks might increase your threat of lung cancer.

Avoiding tobacco — or deciding to stop using it is an important part of cancer prevention. However, ask your croaker
about stop-smoking products and other strategies for quitting, If you need help quitting tobacco.

2. Eat a healthy diet
Although making healthy selections at the grocery store and at mealtime can not guarantee cancer forestallment, it might reduce your threat. Consider these guidelines

Eat plenty of fruits and vegetables. Base your diet on fruits, vegetables, and other foods from factory sources similar to whole grains and sap.
Maintain a healthy weight. Eat lighter and slender by choosing smaller high-calorie foods, including ameliorated sugars and fat from beast sources.
still, do so only in temperance The threat of colorful types of cancer — including cancer of the bone, and colon, If you choose to drink alcohol.
Limit reused flesh. A report from the International Agency for Research on Cancer, the cancer agency of the World Health Organization, concluded that eating large quantities of reused meat can slightly increase the threat of certain types of cancer.
In addition, women who eat a Mediterranean diet supplemented with extra-virgin olive oil painting and mixed nuts might have a reduced threat of bone cancer. The Mediterranean diet focuses substantially on factory-grounded foods, similar to fruits and vegetables, whole grains, legumes, and nuts. People who follow the Mediterranean diet choose healthy fats, similar to olive oil painting, over adulation, and fish rather than red meat.

3. Maintain a healthy weight and be physically active

Maintaining a healthy weight might lower the threat of colorful types of cancer, including cancer of the bone, prostate, lung, colon, and order.

Physical exertion counts, too. In addition to helping you control your weight, physical exertion on its own might lower the threat of bone cancer and colon cancer.

Grown-ups who share in any quantum of physical exertion gain some health benefits. But for substantial health benefits, strive to get at least 150 twinkles a week of moderate aerobic exertion or 75 twinkles a week of vigorous aerobic exertion. You can also do a combination of moderate and vigorous exertion. As a general thing, including at least 30 twinkles of physical exertion in your diurnal routine — and if you can do more, indeed better.

4. cover yourself from the sun
Skin cancer is one of the most common kinds of cancer — and one of the most preventable. Try these tips

Avoid noon sun. Stay out of the sun between 10 a.m. and 4 p.m., when the sun's shafts are strongest.
Stay in the shade. When you are outside, stay in the shade as much as possible. Sunglasses and a broad-brimmed chapeau help, too.
Cover exposed areas. Wear tightly woven, loose befitting apparel that covers as important of your skin as possible. conclude for bright or dark colors, which reflect further ultraviolet radiation than do aquarelles or blanched cotton.
Do not scrimp on sunscreen. Use a broad-diapason sunscreen with an SPF of at least 30, indeed on cloudy days. Apply sunscreen free handedly, and reapply every two hours — or more frequently if you are swimming or perspiring.
Avoid tanning beds and sunlamps. These are just as damaging as the natural sun.

5. Get vaccinated
Cancer forestallment includes protection from certain viral infections. Talk to your croaker
about vaccination against

hepatitis B. Hepatitis B can increase the threat of developing liver cancer. The hepatitis B vaccine is recommended for certain grown-ups at high threat — similar to grown-ups who are sexually active but not in a mutually monogamous relationship, people with sexually transmitted infections, people who use intravenous medicines, men who have coitus with men, and health care or public safety workers who might be exposed to infected blood or body fluids.

mortal papillomavirus(HPV). HPV is a sexually transmitted contagion that can lead to cervical and other genital cancers as well as scaled cell cancers of the head and neck. The HPV vaccine is recommended for girls and boys periods 11 and 12. TheU.S. Food and Drug Administration approved the use of the vaccine Gardasil 9 for males and ladies periods 9 to 45.

6. Avoid parlous actions

Another effective cancer forestallment tactic is to avoid perilous actions that can lead to infections that, in turn, might increase the threat of cancer. For illustration

Practice safe coitus. Limit your number of sexual mates and use a condom when you have coitus. The further sexual mates you have in your continuance, the more likely you're to contract a sexually transmitted infection — similar to HIV or HPV. People who have HIV or AIDS have an advanced threat of cancer of the anus, liver, and lung. HPV is most frequently associated with cervical cancer, but it might also increase the threat of cancer to the anus, penis, throat, vulva, and vagina.

Do not partake of needles. Participating in needles with people who use intravenous medicines can lead to HIV, as well as hepatitis B and hepatitis C — which can increase the threat of liver cancer. However, seek professional help, If you are concerned about medicine abuse or dependence.

7. Get regular medical care

Regular tone- examinations and wireworks for colorful types of cancers similar to cancer of the skin, colon, cervix, and bone — can increase your chances of discovering cancer beforehand, when treatment is most likely to be successful. Ask your croaker about the stylish cancer webbing schedule for you.

About one of every three Americans will develop some form of malice during his or her continuance. Despite these grim statistics, croakers
have made great progress in understanding the biology of cancer cells, and they've formerly been suitable to ameliorate the opinion and treatment of cancer.

But rather than just staying for new improvements, you can do a lot to cover yourself right now. Webbing tests can help describe malice in their foremost stages, but you should always be alert for symptoms of the complaint. The American Cancer Society developed this simple memorial times ago

C Change in bowel or bladder habits
A sore that doesn't heal
U Unusual bleeding or discharge
T Thickening or lump in the bone or away
I have Indigestion or difficulty in swallowing
O egregious change in a nodule or operative
N troubling cough or hoarseness
It's a rough companion that is stylish. The vast maturity of similar symptoms is caused by nonmalignant diseases, and cancers can produce symptoms that do not show up on the list, similar to unexplained weight loss or fatigue. But it's a useful memorial to hear to your body and report sounds of torture to your croaker

.

cover yourself from the damage of habitual inflammation.
Science has proven that habitual, low-grade inflammation can turn into a silent killer that contributes to cardiovas-cular complaints, cancer, type 2 diabetes, and other conditions.
The early opinion is important, but can you go one better? Can you reduce your threat of getting cancer in the first place? It sounds too good to be true, but it's not. Scientists have estimated that up to 75

American cancer deaths can be averted. The 8 commandments of cancer forestallment are

1. Exercise regularly. Physical exertion has been linked to a reduced threat of colon cancer. Exercise also appears to reduce a woman's threat of bone and conceivably reproductive cancers. Exercise will help cover you indeed if you do not lose weight.

2. Stay spare. rotundity increases the threat of numerous forms of cancer. Calories count; if you need to slim down, take in smaller calories and burn more with exercise.

3. still, limit yourself to a normal of one drink a day, If you choose to drink. Redundant alcohol increases the threat of cancers of the mouth, larynx(voice box), esophagus(food pipe), liver, and colon; it also increases a woman's threat of bone cancer. Smoking further increases the threat of numerous alcohol- convinced malice.

4. Avoid gratuitous exposure to radiation. Get medical imaging studies only when you need them. Check your home for domestic radon, which increases the threat of lung cancer. cover yourself from ultraviolet radiation in the sun, which increases the threat of tuberculosis and other skin cancers. But do not worry about electromagnetic radiation from high-voltage power lines or radiofrequency radiation from broilers and cell phones. They don't get cancer.

5. Avoid exposure to artificial and environmental poisons similar to asbestos filaments, benzene, sweet amines, and polychlorinated biphenyls(PCBs).

6. Avoid infections that contribute to cancer, including hepatitis contagions, HIV, and the mortal papillomavirus. numerous are transmitted sexually or through defiled needles.

7. Make quality sleep a priority. Actually, the substantiation linking sleep to cancer isn't strong. But poor and inadequate sleep increases are associated with weight gain, which is a cancer threat factor.

8. Get enough vitamin D. Numerous experts now recommend 800 to,000 IU a day, a thing that is nearly insolvable to attain without taking a supplement. Although protection is far from proven, substantiation suggests that vitamin D may help reduce the threat of prostate cancer, colon cancer, and other malice. But do not count on other supplements.

Chapter 5: Sleep

Sleep Problems in People with Cancer
People going through treatment for cancer may have changes in their sleep patterns or difficulty sleeping. Tell your nanny about any difficulties you're having, so you can get the help you need to sleep better at night.

What sleep problems are common in people being treated for cancer?
Sleep problems similar to being unfit to fall asleep and/ or stay asleep, also called wakefulness, are common among people being treated for cancer.

What causes sleep problems?
Sleep problems may be caused by the side goods of treatment, drugs you're taking, long sanitarium stays, stress, and other factors. Studies show that as numerous as half of all people have sleep-related problems during treatment for cancer.

How are sleep problems assessed?
Your croaker, or a sleep specialist, can do an assessment, which may include a polysomnogram (recordings taken during sleep that show brain swells, breathing rate, and other conditioning similar to heart rate) to diagnose and treat sleep problems. Assessments may be repeated from time to time, since sleeping problems may change over time. Learn further about when a sleep study may be useful,

what to anticipate, and what your croaker may recommend after a sleep study.

Why is a good night's sleep important?
Sleeping well is important for your physical and internal health. A good night's sleep may help you to relax more easily, lower your blood pressure, help your appetite, and strengthen your vulnerable system. Sleep problems that go on for a long time may increase the threat of anxiety or depression.

Talk with your health care platoon if you have difficulty sleeping, so you can get the help you need. There is a way that you and your health care platoon can take to help you sleep well again.

Tell your croaker
about problems that intrude with sleep. Getting treatment to lower problems similar to pain or other side effects similar to urinary and bladder problems, or diarrhea may help you sleep better.
Cognitive behavioral remedies (CBT) and relaxation remedies may help. rehearsing these curatives can help you to relax. For illustration, a CBT therapist can help you learn to change negative studies and beliefs about sleep into positive bones. Strategies similar to muscle relaxation, guided imagery, and tone- hypnotism may also help you.

Set good bedtime habits. Go to bed only when sleepy, in a quiet and dark room, and in a comfortable bed. However, get out of bed and return to bed when you're sleepy, If you don't fall asleep. Stop watching TV or using other electrical bias a couple of hours before going to bed. Don't drink or eat a lot before bedtime. While it's important to keep active during the day with regular exercise, exercising many hours before bedtime may make sleep more delicate.

Sleep drugs may be specified. Your croaker may define sleep drugs, for a short period if other strategies don't work. The sleep drug specified will depend on your specific problem(similar to trouble falling asleep or trouble staying asleep) as well as other drugs you're taking.

Chapter 6: NUTRITION

The anticancer food

Foods That Could Lower Your threat of Cancer
What you eat can drastically affect numerous aspects of your health, including your threat of developing habitual conditions like heart complaints, diabetes, and cancer.
The development of cancer, in particular, has been shown to be heavily told by your diet.
numerous foods contain salutary composites that could help drop the growth of cancer.
There are also several studies showing that an advanced input of certain foods could be associated with a lower threat of the complaint.
This book will claw into the exploration and look at 13 foods that may lower your threat of cancer.

1. Broccoli
Broccoli contains sulforaphane, a factory emulsion set up in cruciferous vegetables that may have potent anticancer parcels.
One test-tube study showed that sulforaphane reduced the size and number of bone cancer cells by over 75%.

Also, a beast study set up that treating mice with sulforaphane helped kill off prostate cancer cells and reduced excrescence volume by further than 50%.

Some studies have also set up that an advanced input of cruciferous vegetables like broccoli may be linked to a lower threat of colorectal cancer. One analysis of 35 studies showed that eating further cruciferous vegetables was associated with a lower threat of colorectal and colon cancer. Including broccoli with many reflections per week may come with some cancer-fighting benefits.

Still, keep in mind that the available exploration hasn't looked directly at how broccoli may affect cancer in humans.

Rather, it has been limited to, test-tube, beast, and experimental studies that either delved the goods of cruciferous vegetables, or the goods of a specific emulsion in broccoli. Therefore, further studies are demanded.

Broccoli contains sulforaphane, an emulsion that has been shown to beget excrescence cell death and reduce excrescence size in test and beast studies. An advanced input of cruciferous vegetables may also be associated with a lower threat of colorectal cancer.

2. Carrots

Several studies have set up that eating further carrots is linked to a dropped threat of certain types of cancer.

For illustration, an analysis looked at the results of five studies and concluded that eating carrots may reduce the threat of stomach cancer by over 26%

Another study set up that an advanced input of carrots was associated with 18 lower odds of developing prostate cancer

One study anatomized the diets of 266 actors with and without lung cancer. It set up that current smokers who didn't eat carrots were three times as likely to develop lung cancer, compared to those who ate carrots further than formerly per week.

Try incorporating carrots into your diet as a healthy snack or succulent side dish just many times per week to increase your input and potentially reduce your threat of cancer.

Still, a flashback shows that these studies show an association between carrot consumption and cancer, but don't account for other factors that may play a part. Some studies have set up an association between carrot consumption and a dropped threat of prostate, lung, and stomach cancer.

3. sap
The sap is high in fiber, which some studies have set up may help cover against colorectal cancer.
One study followed 905 people with a history of colorectal excrescences and set up that those who consumed more cooked, dried sap tended to have a dropped threat of excrescence rush.
A beast study also set up that feeding rats black sap or cortege sap and also converting colon cancer blocked the development of cancer cells by over 75%.
According to these results, eating many servings of sap each week may increase your fiber input and help lower the threat of developing cancer.

Still, the current exploration is limited to beast studies and studies that show association but not the occasion. further studies are demanded to examine this in humans, specifically.
The sap is high in fiber, which may be defensive against colorectal cancer. Mortal and beast studies have set up that an advanced input of sap could reduce the threat of colorectal excrescences and colon cancer.

4. Berries
Berries are high in anthocyanins, factory colors that have antioxidant parcels and may be associated with a reduced threat of cancer.
In one mortal study, 25 people with colorectal cancer were treated with blueberry extract for seven days, which was set up to reduce the growth of cancer cells by 7%.
Another small study gave snap-dried black snorts to cases with oral cancer and showed that it dropped situations of certain labels associated with cancer progression.

One beast study set up that giving rats indurate-dried black snorts reduced esophageal excrescence prevalence by over 54% and dropped the number of excrescences by over 62%.

Also, another beast study showed that giving rats a berry excerpt was set up to inhibit several biomarkers of cancer.

Grounded on these findings, including a serving or two of berries in your diet each day may help inhibit the development of cancer.

Keep in mind that these are beast and experimental studies looking at the goods of a concentrated cure of berry excerpt, and more mortal exploration is demanded.

Some test-tube and beast studies have set up that the composites in berries may drop the growth and spread of certain types of cancer.

5. Cinnamon

Cinnamon is well-known for its health benefits, including its capability to reduce blood sugar and ease inflammation.

In addition, some test-tube, and beast studies have set up that cinnamon may help block the spread of cancer cells.

A test-tube study set up that cinnamon excerpt was suitable to drop the spread of cancer cells and induce their death.

Another test-tube study showed that cinnamon essential oil painting suppressed the growth of head and neck cancer cells, and also significantly reduced excrescence size.

A beast study also showed that cinnamon excerpts convinced cell death in excrescences, and also dropped how important excrescences grew and spread. Including 1/2 – 1 tablespoon(2 – 4 grams) of cinnamon in your diet per day may be salutary in cancer forestallment, and may come with other benefits as well, such as reduced blood sugar and dropped inflammation.

Still, further studies are demanded to understand how cinnamon may affect cancer development in humans.

Test-tube and beast studies have set up that cinnamon excerpts may have anticancer parcels and may help drop the growth and spread of excrescences. further exploration in humans is demanded.

6. Nuts

exploration has set up that eating nuts may be linked to a lower threat of certain types of cancer.

For example, a study looked at the diets of 386 people and set up that eating a lesser quantity of nuts was associated with a dropped threat of dying from cancer.

Another study followed 708 actors over 30 times and set up that eating nuts regularly was associated with a dropped threat of colorectal, pancreatic, and endometrial cancers.

Other studies have set up that specific types of nuts may be linked to a lower cancer threat.

For illustration, Brazil nuts are high in selenium, which may help cover against lung cancer in those with low selenium status.

Also, one beast study showed that feeding mice walnuts dropped the growth rate of bone cancer cells by 80% and reduced the number of excrescences by 60%.

These results suggest that adding a serving of nuts to your diet each day may reduce your threat of developing cancer in the future.

Still, further studies in humans are demanded to determine whether nuts are responsible for this association, or whether other factors are involved. Some studies have set up that increased input of nuts may drop the threat of cancer. exploration shows that some specific types like Brazil nuts and walnuts may also be linked to a lower threat of cancer.

7. Olive Oil

Olive oil painting is loaded with health benefits, so it's no wonder it's one of the masses of the Mediterranean diet.

Several studies have indeed set up that an advanced input of olive oil painting may help cover against cancer.

One massive review made up of 19 studies showed that people who consumed the topmost quantum of olive oil painting had a lower threat of developing bone cancer and cancer of the digestive system than those with the smallest input.

Another study looked at the cancer rates in 28 countries around the world and set up that areas with an advanced input of olive oil painting had dropped rates of colorectal cancer.

switching out other canvases in your diet for olive oil painting is a simple way to take advantage of its health benefits. You can dapple it over salads and cooked vegetables, or try using it in your gravies for meat, fish, or flesh.

Though these studies show that there may be an association between olive oil painting input and cancer, there are likely other factors involved as well. further studies are demanded to look at the direct goods of olive oil painting on cancer in people.

Several studies have shown that an advanced input of olive oil painting may be associated with a reduced threat of certain types of cancer.

8. Turmeric

Turmeric is a spice well-known for its health-promoting parcels. Curcumin, its active component, is a chemical with anti-inflammatory, antioxidant, and indeed anticancer goods.

One study looked at the goods of curcumin in 44 cases with lesions in the colon that could have come cancerous. After 30 days, 4 grams of curcumin daily reduced the number of lesions present by 40%.

In a test-tube study, curcumin was also set up to drop the spread of colon cancer cells by targeting a specific enzyme related to cancer growth.

Another test-tube study showed that curcumin helped kill off head and neck cancer cells.

Curcumin has also been shown to be effective in decelerating the growth of lung, bone, and prostate cancer cells in other test-tube studies.

For stylish results, aim for at least $1/2 - 3$ ladles($1 - 3$ grams) of ground turmeric per day. Use it as a ground spice to add flavor to foods, and brace it with black pepper to help boost its immersion.

Turmeric contains curcumin, a chemical that has been shown to reduce the growth of numerous types of cancer and lesions in test-tubes and mortal studies.

9. Citrus Fruits

Eating citrus fruits similar to failures, limes, grapefruits, and oranges have been associated with a lower threat of cancer in some studies.

One large study set up that actors who ate an advanced quantity of citrus fruits had a lower threat of developing cancers of the digestive and upper respiratory tracts.

A review looking at nine studies also set up that a lesser input of citrus fruits was linked to a reduced threat of pancreatic cancer.

Eventually, a review of 14 studies showed that a high input, or at least three servings per week, of citrus fruit, reduced the threat of stomach cancer by 28%.

These studies suggest that including many servings of citrus fruits in your diet each week may lower your threat of developing certain types of cancer. Studies have set up that an advanced input of citrus fruits could drop the threat of certain types of cancers, including pancreatic and stomach cancers, along with cancers of the digestive and upper respiratory tracts.

10. Flaxseed

High in fiber as well as heart-healthy fats, flaxseed can be a healthy addition to your diet.

Some exploration has shown that it may indeed help drop cancer growth and help kill off cancer cells.

In one study, 32 women with bone cancer entered either a flaxseed muffin daily or a placebo for over a month.

At the end of the study, the flaxseed group had dropped situations of specific labels that measure excrescence growth, as well as an increase in cancer cell death.

In another study, 161 men with prostate cancer were treated with flaxseed, which was set up to reduce the growth and spread of cancer cells.

Flaxseed is high in fiber, which other studies have set up to be defensive against colorectal cancer.

Try adding one teaspoon(10 grams) of ground flaxseed into your diet each day by mixing it into smoothies, sprinkling it over cereal and yogurt, or adding it to your favorite baked goods.

Some studies have set up that flaxseed may reduce cancer growth in bone and prostate cancers. It's also high in fiber, which may drop the threat of colorectal cancer.

11. Tomatoes

Lycopene is an emulsion set up in tomatoes that's responsible for its vibrant red color as well as its anticancer parcels.

Several studies have set up that increased input of lycopene and tomatoes could lead to a reduced threat of prostate cancer.

A review of 17 studies also set up that an advanced input of raw tomatoes, cooked tomatoes, and lycopene were all associated with a reduced threat of prostate cancer.

Another study of 365 people set up that a lesser input of tomato sauce, in particular, was linked to a lower threat of developing prostate cancer.

To help increase your input, include a serving or two of tomatoes in your diet each day by adding them to sandwiches, salads, gravies, or pasta dishes.

Still, a flashback shows that there may be an association between eating tomatoes and a reduced threat of prostate cancer, but they don't account for other factors that could be involved.

Some studies have set up that an advanced input of tomatoes and lycopene could reduce the threat of prostate cancer.

12. Garlic

The active element in garlic is allicin, an emulsion that has been shown to kill off cancer cells in multiple test-tube studies.

Several studies have set up an association between garlic input and a lower threat of certain types of cancer.

One study of 220 actors set up that those who ate lots of Allium vegetables, similar as garlic, onions, leeks, and shallots, had a lower threat of stomach cancer than those who infrequently consumed them.

A study of 471 men showed that an advanced input of garlic was associated with a reduced threat of prostate cancer.

Another study set up that actors who ate lots of garlic, as well as fruit, deep unheroic vegetables, dark green vegetables, and onions, were less likely to develop colorectal excrescences. Still, this study didn't insulate the goods of garlic.

Grounded on these findings, including 2 – 5 grams(roughly one clove) of fresh garlic into your diet per day can help you take advantage of its health-promoting parcels.

Still, despite the promising results showing an association between garlic and a reduced threat of cancer, further studies are demanded to examine whether other factors play a part.

Garlic contains allicin, an emulsion that has been shown to kill cancer cells in test-tube studies. Studies have set up that eating further garlic could lead to dropped pitfalls of stomach, prostate, and colorectal cancers.

13. Adipose Fish

Some exploration suggests that including many servings of fish in your diet each week may reduce your threat of cancer.

One large study showed that an advanced input of fish was associated with a lower threat of digestive tract cancer.

In another study that followed,040 grown-ups stated that eating further fish dropped the threat of developing colorectal cancer, while red and reused flesh actually increased the threat.

In particular, adipose fish like salmon, mackerel, and anchovies contain important nutrients similar to vitamin D and omega- 3 adipose acids that have been linked to a lower threat of cancer.

For illustration, having acceptable situations of vitamin D is believed to cover against and reduce the threat of cancer.

In addition, omega- 3 adipose acids are allowed to block the development of the complaint.

Aim for two servings of adipose fish per week to get a hearty cure of omega- 3 adipose acids and vitamin D, and to maximize the implicit health benefits of these nutrients.

Still, further exploration is demanded to determine how adipose fish consumption may directly impact the threat of cancer in humans.

Fish consumption may drop the threat of cancer. Adipose fish contain vitamin D and omega- 3 adipose acids, two nutrients that are believed to protect against cancer.

In conclusion

As new exploration continues to crop, it has come increasingly clear that your diet can have a major impact on your threat of cancer.

Although there are numerous foods that have the potential to reduce the spread and growth of cancer cells, current exploration is limited to test-tube, beast, and experimental studies.

further studies are demanded to understand how these foods may directly affect cancer development in humans.

In the meantime, it's a safe bet that a diet rich in whole foods, paired with a healthy life, will ameliorate numerous aspects of your health.